The Art of
GIVING BIRTH

The Art of
GIVING BIRTH

With Chanting,
Breathing, and Movement

FRÉDÉRICK LEBOYER, M.D.
TRANSLATED BY ARIEL GODWIN

Healing Arts Press
Rochester, Vermont

Healing Arts Press
One Park Street
Rochester, Vermont 05767
www.HealingArtsPress.com

Healing Arts Press is a division of Inner Traditions International

Originally published in German under the title *Atmen, singen, gebären* by Patmos Verlag
    GmbH & Co. KG
First U.S. edition published in 2009 by Healing Arts Press under the title *The Art of
    Giving Birth*

*Note to the reader: This book is intended as an informational guide. The remedies,
approaches, and techniques described herein are meant to supplement, and not to be a
substitute for, professional medical care or treatment. They should not be used to treat a
serious ailment without prior consultation with a qualified health care professional.*

Library of Congress Cataloging-in-Publication Data
Leboyer, Frédérick.
   [Atmen, singen, gebären. English]
   The art of giving birth : with chanting, breathing, and movement / Frédérick Leboyer ;
translated by Ariel Godwin.
      p. cm.
   "Originally published in German under the title: Atmen, singen, gebären, by Patmos
Verlag GmbH & Co., c2006."
   ISBN 978-1-59477-276-4 (pbk.)
   1. Natural childbirth. I. Title.
   RG661.L3813
   618.4'5—dc22

                                                            2008041958

Printed and bound in the United States at Lake Book Manufacturing

10   9   8   7   6   5   4   3   2   1

Text design and layout by Virginia Scott Bowman
This book was typeset in Garamond Premier Pro with Schneidller Initials, Gil Sans, and
Cochin Italic as display typefaces

To send correspondence to the author of this book, mail a first-class letter to the author
c/o Inner Traditions • Bear & Company, One Park Street, Rochester, VT 05767, and we
will forward the communication.

Contents

∞

PART TWO

The Art of Breathing and Singing

∞

Foreword

Dear Frédérick,

As you know, I was deeply affected when I read your first book, *Birth without Violence*,* more than twenty-five years ago. It was a determining influence in my professional development and my life. I made the decision to become a midwife so that, as a woman, I could help other women in this regard.

Today I am writing to you again, since my everyday work is so discouraging. All women—and I really do mean all—don't want to hear a word about giving birth without peridural anesthesia. But with this, they not only miss out on the greatest and most important experience in a woman's life but also show no awareness of the extremely harmful side effects this kind of interference can have. What's more, these effects are rarely explained to them.

You have said that you are working on a new book to

Birth without Violence was first published in French in 1974.

show women how they can make giving birth the most beautiful, glorious day of their lives, including statements from numerous women who have been lucky enough to use alternative methods for giving birth. Never has such a book been more urgently needed. When will it be published? And when will it be translated?

On my own behalf, and on behalf of all women, I thank you for the work you have done.

MARTA CAMPIOTI,
CHAIR OF THE ITALIAN NATIONAL
OBSTETRIC ORGANIZATION FOR
HOME BIRTHS AND BIRTHING CENTERS
VARESE, ITALY

PART ONE

Giving Birth
with the Help of Tai Chi
and the Tambūrā

When we are born, we cry, that we are come
To this great stage of fools.

SHAKESPEARE, *KING LEAR*

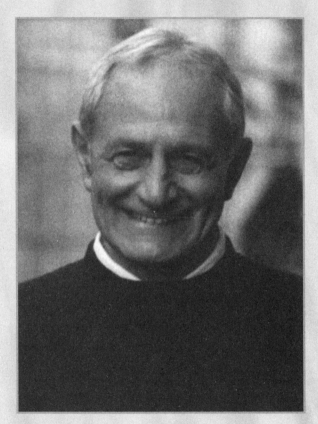

Frédérick Leboyer

To Lisa Who Is Having a Baby

∞

(A Letter from Frédérick Leboyer)

Dear Lisa,

Thank you for your wonderful letter, telling me that you are expecting a baby. Please accept my congratulations!

You also tell me that a friend gave you my first book, *Birth without Violence,* and that after reading it, full of exaltation, you cried out: "Yes! That's the way I want to give birth!" And then you asked me for the address of a hospital or birthing clinic or the name of a doctor, or midwife, who uses these methods. I hope you will not be upset with me when I tell you that I think you may not have read and understood my book correctly. Rather than giving you

3

names and addresses, I would like to offer you my own help and show you what you have misunderstood. Allow me to explain further.

You've become a little confused, but it isn't entirely your fault. Childbirth is something ambivalent. It is like a medal or a coin, showing one side but actually having two. Allow me to explain this, too.

At the end of her pregnancy, a woman goes into labor and finally brings a baby into the world. The term for this is "giving birth." When speaking of the child, we say that it "comes into the world." This means that it is "born"—and as you can see, it's an extraordinary experience on both sides. There is the experience of the woman, bringing a child into the world; and there is the experience of the child, leaving its mother and being thrown into a world so different that it will never recover from the shock.

For consider this: although everyone knows that childbirth can be one of the most painful experiences in a woman's life, before the publication of my book *Birth without Violence* nobody ever asked whether being born, for a baby, might be just as painful and frightening as giving birth is for the mother. But indeed, contrary to earlier ideas, the baby does "experience" its birth, its arrival in the world; even well before birth, it "already" has consciousness and perceptions, and even a pronounced sense of justice, so that it must wonder: "Why? Why this, then? What did I do to be thrown out the door of this paradise, the mother's womb?" Will the baby be thrown out the door, or will it feel more as if its time has come to set out on its journey? This is the subject of *Birth without Violence*.

You see, this is all about the drama the child experiences when it is born—not at all about what people call "childbirth." In other words: when a newborn is *somebody* and not just *something*—when he or she is a person, and not merely a *condition*—then everything is different. A condition afflicts one, requires treatment, and is not something friendly. But with a *person*, we deal in an entirely different way. We show the person some consideration.

In German, there is a beautiful expression that describes the situation very well: a woman doesn't say that she's "had" a baby, but that she's "received" a baby. Like a gift or a visit. And what a visit! A visit from a prince!

So, once again: my book *Birth without Violence* is only about the baby's experience. Not a word about what the woman goes through during childbirth. Many women were quite annoyed. "This Leboyer," they said, "he only cares about the child. Our suffering doesn't matter to him in the least."

Of course it *does* matter to me! I did not speak of it in that book for two reasons: firstly, because I was so fascinated, so absorbed by—if I may call it this—"my discovery." Namely, I had realized that "being born" is awful and scary for the child. Now I had to find out how this newly arrived baby, who ought to be radiating joy since it is no longer imprisoned, might heal from its perturbation. It should be transported by happiness, instead of meeting its arrival in the world with obvious anguish and fear. This was such a fantastic discovery that I could only compare it with the first time someone ever planted a seed in the earth and nurtured it to grow. This was the person who discovered agriculture. And here I was, discovering how a child could be born joyfully, without suffering.

The other reason I said nothing about the woman's pain, or how she could be spared it, was that at the time I knew nothing about it. I also believed (and how wrong I was!) that the answer had already been found by those people who advertised what they deceptively called "painless birth," trying to make women believe that they could give birth without feeling a thing. But with their methods, giving birth is like an earthquake, a tidal wave, a hurricane. It can be an exciting adventure—for those who can hold onto the rudder.

Meaning to say, it is not possible for a woman to give birth without feeling anything. But what she feels can be a great joy to her. Before I say more on this topic—which is the actual subject of this book—let's take another look at the false ideas that you, like so many other women, have about giving birth.

Listen carefully, now. What you're about to learn will shock you!

Who can eat for you? Nobody, obviously.

Who can sleep for you? Also nobody.

And who can give birth for you? Nobody. Nobody but you, you, you!

Once you have come to terms with this fundamental fact, all your problems will be solved, and you will finally stop trying to figure out whom, in what place, will give birth for you. And you will understand that you only have to do one thing: stand by yourself.

Where do these erroneous ideas come from, that someone can give birth for someone else? Partly, they come from the idea that you are not the one giving birth. The birth and the labor contractions are beyond your control. It will happen within you of its own accord, and you will merely observe it, like the digestion of food you eat. But the observer can either acquiesce with events, or do the opposite and resist them, mobilizing all her power against them. We will return to this.

There is another fundamental idea, hitherto completely ignored: if you are not the one giving birth for yourself, if you are only an observer of the process taking place in you, this means that the child—yes, the child—has to make his own effort to be born. It has been scientifically proven that the signals for birth come from the child's body; the child emits the hormones that bring on labor. The child makes the greatest exertion to be born. You are merely there to help.

In other words, birth is experienced on both sides. That is the revolutionary approach of my first book.

But let us return to these false beliefs that so many women have about childbirth, and to how they picture birth.

Is this baby who is going to be born out of you something

like a bad tooth that needs to be pulled out? Are you therefore looking for a good dentist?

Pulled out—the way one opens a wine bottle with a corkscrew? Note the image is not so incongruous. The womb containing the baby is shaped like an amphora: a bulging container with a small opening, stopped up not with a cork but with a mucous membrane that disintegrates all by itself to let the baby through. Does one need a corkscrew for that? For wine, sure, but what if we're drinking . . . champagne?

When this life suddenly breaks out, positively exploding and frothing all over like some heavenly drink, what use is a corkscrew?

You must realize that a birth is like an explosion of joy. Life surges up in you, so strong that it breaks all limits, all barriers. It is like a river rising so high that it engulfs and sweeps away everything in its path.

What is it that "floods" over everything at a birth? It is life! It is love! And yes, it is joy! And all this has so much strength that it can frighten and overwhelm you.

There is a name for the flooded banks of the river that rush beyond all control: they are the "little I," or if you prefer, your ego, which could not possibly have imagined an experience of such magnitude. And when this little I feels itself being pulled along with the current, it digs its heels in and resists. The same reaction takes place in psychoanalysis, which also involves so much resistance.

There is an answer to the question "where to give birth?"—wherever your labor pains begin. And if you're at the supermarket, head home as soon as possible. "Where should I go? Who will give birth for me?" All these questions will disappear once you understand that nobody, nobody at all can give birth for you.

Unfortunately, the little I, the ego, does not give up so easily. The resistances form themselves into words: "Give birth at home? Is that wise? Isn't that running a great risk?" Since (as you know or at least suspect) this is the fear talking, the whole hocus-pocus starts over again from the beginning: "Am I not exposing my child to a great deal of danger?" No question about it! Anyone you ask will send you straight to a doctor, and then you are trapped, fallen into the pit:

ॐ

"Doctor, I'm expecting a baby."
　"Yes?"
　"And I . . .".
　"You're afraid?"
　"Yes, Doctor, you guessed it."
　"So, fear. A little bit of fear?"
　"No, to be honest, I'm terrified."

ॐ

So the obstetrician takes things in hand.

"You shouldn't be ashamed. Your fear is entirely natural. Childbirth is a high-risk condition, with many dangers."

"Is it really?"

"Yes. Also, this is all new for you."

"That must be why I'm afraid?"

"Of course."

"Doctor, since you know so much and I know nothing, absolutely nothing, will you give birth for me?"

"Very gladly."

"My friend who gave me your address told me you sedated her [or gave her peridural or epidural anesthesia] when she gave birth. Will you do that with me as well?"

"You can depend on me, I promise."

"Ah, Doctor, how can I thank you? I'm so relieved and reassured."

And so the woman has fallen into a quite ingenious snare.

Why does she fall into it? Because of her fear, obviously. This fear is the secret lever for all power mechanisms, whether their power is political, religious, or in this case, medical.

Since those in power have mutually assisted one another, we have arrived at the present state of things: women do not feel empowered to give birth themselves, and they exclude the possibility for reasons of safety. But there has never been safety; life simply *is* risky, all the time, everywhere, including during childbirth. Giving birth is a leap into the unknown, and any "sensible" woman must find such a thing extremely exciting—but for sure, it is quite a change from the dreary monotony of everyday.

Is childbirth really all that dangerous? Not at all! Is it all that risky? No, it's the most natural thing there is. Is it all that scary? Well, yes.

But fear and danger are not the same thing. Perhaps you know the story of the rope and the snake. A man is walking along a path. Suddenly he stops: There! A snake! He is petrified—until he notices that the snake isn't moving. He steps forward, edges toward it very cautiously. The "snake" is just a piece of rope. Why did he make the mistake? Fear, of course.

There's an important question here: why do the obstetricians behave the way they do? Is it the lure of money? Do they want to take credit for the births? Sometimes. But these are not the deciding factors. Much more so, they believe childbirth is full of risks.

Where does this false belief come from? It comes from the fact that these obstetricians had traumatic births themselves. The unconscious memory of this unpleasant beginning of their lives is engraved in the depths of their innermost consciousness and has dictated their choice of career, in which, quite obsessively, they can experience again and again the pain of the scars they bear. Also, most obstetricians are men. How could they leave such an important event as the birth of a child up to *women*, whose brains are so inferior to theirs? Here we find the oldest battle in the world: the battle of the sexes! Even such an intelligent man as the great Aristotle could not accept the idea that the most important role in childbirth is the role of the woman, the mother, rather than that of the man, the father. In his view, the woman was merely the soil in which the seed was planted and grew.

$\sim$

Are danger and fear the same? Not at all, although they are so closely connected. And so it is wrong for obstetricians (even with the best intentions) to stir up a woman's fears, rather than assuaging them, when they warn her not to give birth without their supervision. The following is a proof of my claim. Pay close attention!

In Germany, in the city of Münster, there is a midwife who has just celebrated her three thousandth home birth. Her name, I will gladly tell you, is Raphaela Hoyer.

Here is her story:

At the age of seventeen, she read *Birth without Violence* and made the decision: she would become a midwife. She went through her training, and when she had her diploma, she worked in the birthing center of a local hospital. There, under the direction of her supervisor, she gave birth to her first child. This experience was so catastrophic that afterward, she made an irreversible decision: Never again! Not for me, not for other women! From that day on, she did only home births.

After she had attended my tai chi chuan movements,* she used these techniques in the births of her other three children and helped pregnant women to prepare. Instead of giving birth for them, she accompanied them through giving birth. None of these births were completely painless, but all were full of joy! Although she has now assisted over three thousand women in giving birth, just recently celebrating this milestone, there have been fewer than ten caesarian sections in her twenty-five years of work. And almost all these women have given birth without episiotomies and without tearing. This includes babies weighing five kilograms (11 pounds) at birth.

I should also mention that the women didn't have to lie down on the ghastly birthing table—which, in fact, is only useful for gynecological surgery, for example, after a perineal rupture. With Raphaela, the women naturally go down on all fours and give birth crouching, giving them more control over the whole course of events.

This ridiculous practice of making women give birth lying on their backs has been in place for a long time, without anyone questioning why. Even in the olden days, when everyone still gave birth at home, women would be made to lie down on their backs, on freshly cleaned kitchen towels. But it is absolutely necessary to crouch.

---

*Singing to the sound of the tambūrā will be explained in part 2 of this book. The tambūrā (or tanpūrā) is a stringed instrument used in India for continuous bass drones. One does not actually play melodies on it, but rather an unceasing C G C drone (in Sanskrit, *sa pa sa*): the perfect chord, the symbol of universal harmony.

ℐ

Dear Lisa, now I will share a secret with you that will help you more than anything else to understand where one should give birth, and where not. This secret remained hidden from me for many years.

I had brought more than nine thousand children into the world (that is how I used to describe it, as obstetricians generally do) before I noticed—discovered—that giving birth, for a woman, is the high point, the crowning moment, of her sex life. This seems so obvious, doesn't it?

Yes, giving birth is so closely connected, has so many similarities, with pleasuring yourself. The same slow forward movement, the same pauses, the same gathering of momentum. . . . And anyone with a good ear can tell you that the sounds, tones, and breathing of a woman giving birth and a woman nearing orgasm are the same.

If you don't believe me, then listen to what Professor E. Ph., one of the most highly recognized obstetricians, perhaps the most renowned in Great Britain, has to say:

> A young girl was seduced by her uncle. (Freud would call this father transference!) She became pregnant. Forced to hide her shame, she decided to give birth on the other side of the English Channel.
>
> Arriving in London, where she knew no one, she found a small hotel and took a room there. She felt herself to be in a good situation, not exposed to indiscreet

eyes, and she began to have labor pains that same evening, and gave birth all alone. Her only concern was that she didn't want to wake up the people in the neighboring room. She went through labor entirely guided by instinct. When the moment came, she squeezed while crouching over a wastebasket she had covered with a towel. And so the baby came out. The placenta followed naturally.

At the birthing center she went to after the birth, they asked her, "Didn't you have great pains? Didn't it hurt you?"

She replied: "Hurt me? Oh yes, of course; just a little. About . . . about just the same as I felt when I went to bed with my boyfriend, for the first time."

A bit painful, certainly, but also what bliss, what joy!

Professor E. Ph. adds that this young woman was very lucky to have gotten through this all by herself. It was indeed a miracle. But that is not true. It was nothing unusual. And this man could not grasp that idea. This finely perceptive gentleman was unable to accept that this fundamental act of giving birth could be left up to a creature who, although not entirely contemptible, was certainly inferior to a man in any case. A woman, whose brain is known to be smaller than a man's, less developed, etc. etc., a silly wench, cannot be trusted to give birth on her own.

I can still hear him saying, "No, really, one can't let women give birth alone. Not all alone, without us, without our help!"

But if giving birth is obviously the crowning point of your sex life, the triumph of Eros, then what is the point of anesthesia and sedatives, designed to stop you from feeling anything?

A young English lady who was not in the least prepared for her wedding night supposedly cried out the following: "Please, milord, in or out! But prithee, stop with this foolish back and forth!"

Would a young woman call out for her mother during her first time?

I will stop here. When discussing sexuality, one is treading on risky territory.

ℐ

Dear Lisa, what else should I tell you?

Quite concretely, one can summarize by saying that a woman giving birth has two enemies. But fundamentally, there is only one: her posture, namely the great tendency toward the hollow back.

Her heavy belly pulls her forward, and she reacts to this with an unnaturally thrust-out back. The result of this excessive bending is weak, shallow breathing in the upper chest only. You should aim to breathe strongly, from your abdomen, and work on being able to breathe this way without thinking about it. But this will be discussed more extensively later in this book.

Next, let us proceed to the fatal hollow back.

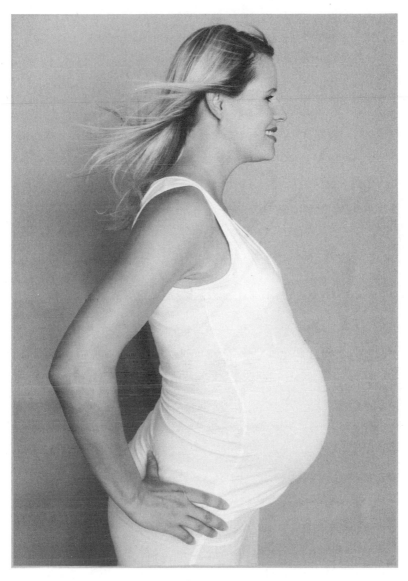

THE BACK

OH, THIS HOLLOW BACK! THIS HOLLOW BACK!

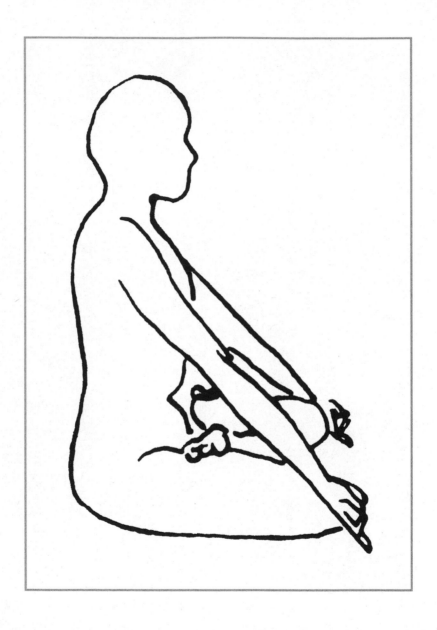

Straightness?
Yes, that is the right word.

Straight, but not rigid!
Flexible, in harmony with the situation.

A straight back?
Of course!
Bolt upright, as they say

A straightened back? A corrected posture?
Corrected, yes, but not under pressure!

A strong back, not a wooden plank!

Body and soul are participating equally,
are one.

Confucius.

Body and mind?
Body and soul?

No!
The two are only one:
The two sides of one and the same coin!

⁒

Has all I have said to you persuaded you that giving birth can be an experience of pure joy? I am not sure myself. There are too many errors and misunderstandings in this topic, even leading to a complete misinterpretation of holy scripture: "In sorrow thou shalt bring forth children" (Genesis 3:16) is a shameful mistranslation. "In sorrow"? No! What was written was more like: "You will have to exert yourself to bring forth children"!

Exertion, hard work, and labor are not the same as sorrow and suffering. "Work! Exert yourselves! Therein will be your greatest reward."* Didn't Jean de la Fontaine say that? Is exertion the same thing as suffering? No, not at all.

Giving birth doesn't just happen; no one would argue with that. It can't happen without some effort. Think of the way we say: "May I trouble you for some advice?" Does "trouble" here mean "hurt" or "injure"? That would be absurd.

To get to the awkward point: can a woman have an orgasm while she is thinking of something else—while watching television, for example? Of course not, she must—yes, *must*—concentrate entirely. Don't forget, we're on the same terrain here.

And just to convince you, I invite you to read and think over what women have written to me after attending my seminars and then giving birth joyously.

---

*"Travaillez, prenez de la peine. C'est le fonds qui manque le moins." From Jean de la Fontaine, *Le laboureur et ses enfants* (The Laborer and His Children).

Zen in the
Art of Giving Birth

∞

Letters from Women

Beata B., Budapest

During the preparations for so-called "painless" birthing, women are told what they should do and what they should not do, how their husbands can provide support, and so forth.

What people forget to tell them—what nobody ever tells them—is that giving birth is an immense, intense experience, an entirely personal experience, in which the woman does not feel lonely or abandoned, but simply alone. Alone like never before. Absolutely alone, yet entirely suffused with an energy that she has never dreamed of before. It is a moment of great intimacy for her.

Doctors and women alike try to make each other believe that the woman can be helped by others. That is wrong, entirely wrong. I would like to testify to this. Help, the only real kind of help, can only come from oneself, and from no one else. I can also attest to that.

As for fear: yes, I am still afraid when I am expecting a child, even very afraid. But I have learned to be courageous. One simply has to stare the fear in the face, then it disappears on the spot. It also helps me to know that I am free, entirely free. I expect no help from outside. By now, in fact, I know that such help simply doesn't exist. I can, and want to, rely only on myself.

Support from my husband? All I expect from him is that he should shield me, guaranteeing me complete calm. Because when this calm is lacking, how can I concentrate on myself and on what is going on inside me?

When labor contractions set in, a woman is extremely sensitive. The slightest discord—a slammed door, a shrill voice, a jangling object being dropped—is like being stabbed for her. I ask my husband to shield me from these things.

The most important thing in pregnancy is for the woman to remain continuously—and I really mean without any interruption—in connection with her child. How can she form this contact? It is simple: she just needs quiet. The woman should sit alone in a space where no one will disturb her. If necessary she should shut the doors, and then listen to her child. She should not try to listen to the noises the child makes in her; as far as it is possible, she should stop thinking about anything. Things must be completely quiet in her.

And what a surprise! It is as if the woman is learning something from her baby. But it is not information, not at all. It is more as if the woman begins to feel that she knows everything worth knowing. And then how can there be fear? There will be no question of that any longer. She will enjoy this calm and this inner peace.

❧ *Commentary*

What a letter! How beautiful! And everything said in it is so profound.

Lisa, dear Lisa, read this letter, read it again and again! You will learn everything from it that one can learn from life. And you will also be freed from the fear that afflicts and constricts all of us—yes, indeed, all of us.

Martina H., Vöcklamarkt

Dear Mr. Leboyer,

In June 1998 my first child, Maximilian-Raphael, came into the world, eight weeks after I met you in Rattenberg, Austria, and attended your seminar, learning the tai chi chuan exercises and singing the notes to the sound of the tambūrā.

After the birth of my son, I wrote to you to thank you and share my astonishment with you. I told you that in the last weeks before giving birth, I had the courage to look my fear in the face, right in the eyes, and that lo and behold, this fear was no longer there. After that, there was only an ocean of life and love.

Late last year, right before the new millennium, I felt the desire for a second child. In fact, I became pregnant soon afterward. Since I was so confident, my pregnancy went by brilliantly, without the least fear. I trusted in my own body, myself, and in what would come out of me.

Three months before the birth we spent ten days on Rhodes. There, on the beach, I once again began the tai chi: the inner work that was my preparation for giving birth.

Of course the child would be born at home. Only the father, a midwife, and a very close friend of mine would be present.

Two weeks before the birth, I had a feeling of great closeness between the baby and myself. It was as if I could feel it pushing downward, coming closer and closer to earth.

Three days before the birth, I experienced something

else, both beautiful and strange. I was lying down to rest on the couch, when it suddenly became clear to me: the baby that was going to be born was . . . me! Yes—it was as if I myself were coming into the world. At these thoughts, my eyes filled with tears. How I cried! What an incomprehensible, but at the same time unforgettable, experience!

On Sunday I had contractions all day long, so I got the room ready for the birth. I set up candles and burned incense. But the midwife I had called—an old, very wise woman—said to me: "No, it's not time yet. I'll come back again in two days."

As I meditated on this, it seemed to me as if the child was telling me it still wanted to wait a while. And indeed, the contractions began again two days later. The candles were lit, and I took a nice warm bath with lavender added to it. As I lay in the water, several fairly loud tones began to come out of me.* I had been in the tub less than half an hour when I sensed that I absolutely had to get out of the water. So I lay down on my couch. I felt a powerful energy. But I could tell that this energy wasn't able to leave my body, as it ought to. I paced up and down the room so that the energy could circulate in me. And all at once there came a strong tone (how strong it was!), and the energy left my body, through my feet.

This energy, as strong as the contractions themselves, seemed to come from above in a waveform and to flow

---

*Here, Martina is talking about singing the tones *A, E, O, I, U, M*. See part 2 of this book.

right through me, then straight down into the earth. I was surprised by the strength and power of these contractions, these waves. Yes, they were waves, following thick and fast one after the other. The first time I had given birth, these waves had been considerably gentler. Now they felt like fire. Yes, they were fire waves—what power, and what violence!

But the tone was there—like a surfboard. This deep, solemn tone, this *O*, this *A*. Thanks to the tone, I could glide over the terrible, violent, energy-laden waves. The tones freed me from all pain, all anguish. I felt the contractions, the waves, coming and giving the tones their pitch. They were so strong, they were my lifeboat. The whole time, the sound of the tambūrā accompanied me. The midwife was there, too, but she kept herself, and all her wisdom about the secret of birth, in the background. It may seem strange, but I had the impression that all existing knowledge about this oracle—for indeed, the arrival of a baby is an oracle—was present in the room with me.

An even larger and more intense wave came over me, and I had to breathe in new air and start the tone again, since I had sustained it so long. Then I turned my attention to the child and asked it for a breather. I also turned off the tambūrā. Now I had to rest; I needed silence. I lay back down on my couch. Ah, what a deep, prolonged rest. It felt as if those waves would never roll over me again. The midwife looked at me and said: "The first stage of the birth is over. Now your cervix is open." This is the opening of the womb. A long, long resting pause followed.

Then new contractions and waves came over me, but they were much less strong. Suddenly the amniotic sac burst. I quickly sat on a birthing chair but immediately knew it wasn't right for me. And then I found myself involuntarily on all fours! This was perfect, just how it was meant to be. All at once I felt as if the baby was "rounding the last bend." I could feel how quickly it was on its way. The midwife was warning me: "Slowly! Slowly!" but how could I listen to her? I couldn't hear anything anymore. With the last wave, the child was born.

I embraced him with both hands and laid him on myself—I was lying on my back by now—and covered him with both hands to keep him warm, to protect him, to soothe him, to take any fear away from him. We waited until the umbilical cord stopped pulsing before we cut it. And at that same exact moment, the child took in a deep breath, without fear and without the least pain. I held him to my breast, and together we took a nice warm bath. Then he fell asleep.

Julian is his name, and now he is three months old. What a wonderful child! So far I haven't had the least problem with him: no colic, no crying. He smiles and smiles and smiles. In fact, he shines with total joy; he radiates calm and happiness.

PS:

Dear Mr. Leboyer,

I urge you to tell women—to tell all women—that it really is possible to bring a child into the world without suffering, without the least pain, without the least anguish, but rather in joy. May your pioneering efforts be successful and lead to the well-being of all future mothers and their children.

May heaven bless you!

I want to add one more thing:

Birth without pain? Without suffering? Not entirely, but I must explain this more exactly.

When I had my first child—before then, I had already attended your seminar—the first part of the labor, the dilation stage, was entirely wonderful, thanks to the singing and the tambūrā. Then nothing else happened. Everything was quiet for two hours—long enough for me to fall asleep. At no time was I fearful or impatient. And yet, at some point, I thought: No, this isn't right.

So what did I do, and what was done to me? An injection? Pituitary extract? Nothing of the kind. I turned my mind toward my baby and said to him: "Now listen to me. It's time. It's been long enough. You can't stay in me any longer. That's over. Your hour has come. You must leave me. Now is your time to come into the world. Do you understand me? Out! Go away! Leave me! Right now! Yes, go, go already!"

The answer was immediate. The contractions came back, and a few minutes later my baby was there.

Did the contractions cause me pain? None at all. But the fact that I had to tell the child with whom I had lived so long, with whom I had shared everything and been so happy,

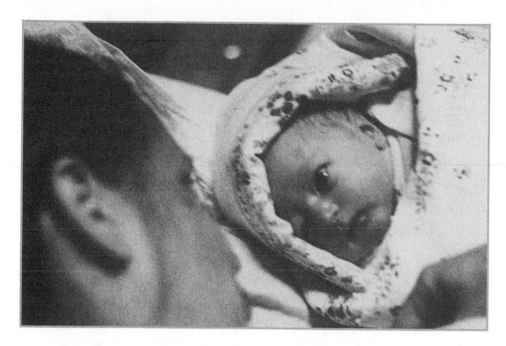

in a commanding tone: "Go, get out, leave me! Your hour is here, you must leave me, do you understand? Come out, leave already!"—this almost tore my heart apart. It was like losing everything.

But as soon as the child was born, we were just like two lovers. We looked into each other's eyes, and all worry was forgotten in a flash, leaving room for other things. . . .

❧ *Commentary*

What more is there to say? What a letter, what a magnificent report!

Here, all the mistakes women normally make when giving birth are avoided and replaced by exactly the right steps:

1. Don't lie in bed once the contractions have set in. In regular clinics, women are put into bed as soon as they come in, as if they are sick. But instead, you should walk up and down, pace around a lot, and not just in any old way. You should not wear shoes, not even slippers or house shoes, and no socks, but instead walk with bare feet. This way, a message is transferred through your feet. All the meridians of acupuncture start in your feet. And you should be sure to connect walking and breathing harmonically with each other: take a step, then breathe out with a tone!

2. Once the contractions have reached a certain strength, the woman can stop walking. She should sit down, but not just any way; she should sit upright, but without stiffening. And then, listening to the sound of the tambūrā, she should move with the tones.

   How should she sit? In half-lotus position if she has done yoga, but never right on the floor. Otherwise her knees may stick up, not making contact with the earth. Sit in the half-lotus position on a firm cushion, preferably a Japanese zafu.

   She can sit in Japanese style, with her heels against her buttocks. In this case there should be a light pillow between them.

   Or she can simply sit on a chair, better yet a simple stool, so that she won't lean back.

3. Between the two stages of birth, everything should be quiet. No tambūrā. Nothing. Complete, absolute quiet.

4. How should she bear down? Never! Never again in the way it still is so often done on the infamous birthing table, where the woman lies on her back and is therefore in no position to bear down, leaving her helpless like a tortoise or a beetle flipped over on its back. Anyone who has taken a couple of judo lessons knows that you're lost as soon as someone has you on your back.

   So, on all fours! The obstetricians hate this, because it injures their pride. . . .

5. The tambūrā should be playing throughout the first stage. The woman will bring forth her own tones as an echo of this tone. This is absolutely not a matter of singing.*

6. As for the bath, and this new, ridiculous craze for giving birth in water, Martina obviously sensed very quickly that she had to get out of the tub. Why? Because the storm and its terrible waves are a storm of electromagnetic fields that surround the body. Palpable changes occur within their range. Some people call this the "subtle body" or the aura. In any case, water hinders and blocks these energies. As the work of William Reich showed, the woman does feel a certain lightness when she is in the water.

---

*See part 2 for a closer explanation of this technique.

This is because her chest breathing changes to diaphragm breathing. But she is lying horizontally, and her feet have lost that all-important contact with the earth.

The vogue for giving birth in water is absurd. That's probably why it is so widespread. During the entire dilation stage the woman should pace up and down, walk, and not hang onto a handhold or onto her husband's neck. Her feet must be on the ground! And the style of walking should be the same style practiced in Japanese martial arts and in Zen meditation.

7. A final remark of great importance: Martina tells us she had a strange experience three days before the birth. While stretched out on the couch, she felt that the baby that was about to come into the world was herself. It was as if she was experiencing her own birth. . . .

Yvonne Fitzgerald, my resourceful English translator for *Birth without Violence*, described what she experienced as follows: "As soon as the contractions set in, the woman enters a different state of consciousness. It's as if she's on another planet. Even time isn't the same as it was before, and she stops pacing and stands still. The woman finds herself in an eternal presence. Everything seems to have fallen apart: past, present, future. And then, she suddenly has the feeling of being simultaneously the mother giving birth and the child being born. She is standing beyond a barrier where all boundary lines and all differences have vanished. Being born and dying are the same thing, indeed there are no more borders, only a single door through which one comes in and goes out. All this is rather confusing."

Birth without Violence has a great deal of information for a woman soon to give birth. But this book is not about obstetrics, and certainly not about any method.

Christiana B., Florence

Dear Dr. Leboyer,

Finally I have found the time to write to you and tell you how my son Martino was born.

But first, I would like to tell you that this birth was the richest and most beautiful experience of my life. And all that I learned from you during the seminar in Pisa was an incalculable help to me.

From that day on, I devoted myself unceasingly to what I had learned there. Every morning I went into my room, got in a good sitting position—just as I'd been taught—and began to sing, or rather, I practiced the tone, accompanied by the sound of the tambūrā on the *Breathing and Singing* tape.* I trained, so to speak, to master the contractions when the time came for them. And so at the end of my pregnancy I was disposed to be very relaxed, calm, and even jovial. At the same time, though, I was anxious and curious to finally meet this child. Perhaps I was even more curious as to whether I would be able to stand up to these fundamental, atavistic pains, so much talked and written about.

The "alarm contractions," if one may call them that, set in on April 25. I felt them all day long. In the evening I was taken to the hospital. They hooked me up to an electronic fetal monitor. The doctor told me my cervix had dilated to

---

*Christiana is referring to the now out-of-print *Atmen und Singen. Einführung, Übungen. Mit einer Übungskassette von Savitry Nayr und Frédérick Leboyer zur "Kunst zu atmen"* (Munich: Kösel, 1984). The lessons contained therein are presented in a revised and simplified form in part 2 of the present book.

three centimeters. But since it was my first birth, this could last as long as twenty-four hours. So she recommended that I go back home. I said I would rather stay in the clinic—and before I had even brushed my teeth to go to bed, I felt two extremely strong twinges in my belly: the amniotic sac had burst.

From this moment on, I fell into a kind of trance, which lasted until the birth was over. Time and space no longer existed for me. How long did the dilation stage last? I have no idea. My husband told me later that the complete cervical dilation was reached in only two hours. I had asked that my husband, who had driven back home, should be informed so that he could come back to me immediately.

So I was in a trance, and I found myself on all fours in a huge bed. There was nothing beyond myself and these limitless pains. In English one would call them "devastating"; another good word might be "destroying." There were no boundaries, resistance was futile, and they rolled over me unrelentingly without giving me a moment to breathe.

At the same time, I was inwardly determined to experience everything entirely consciously. So during the whole dilation stage, I breathed out with a tone every time. Again and again, the *A* and *O* tones came from my mouth, just as I had learned: mouth wide open, eyes closed, my partner's hand in mine.

It was as if the tone was pervading my entire being. My whole body vibrated. This tone seemed to envelop the waves, to absorb the contractions breaking over me. My mind—

indeed, my entire attention—was directed to this tone, and this made me able to grab onto each contraction, each wave flowing over me, and to flow with it, riding the tiger as it were, experiencing everything that was occurring in full consciousness.

I was entirely aware, then, and I felt like a witness to what was going on inside me. But if my concentration wavered—if I thought of anything else, even for a split second—then I was no longer the witness but only a deplorable wreck, tossed up and down by the waves. I could no longer be helped, I was about to go under for the last time, and in the next instant I would find my death in the waves. This is what happened when my total attention was no longer directed to the tone but to the suffering, the pains, which now became unbearable, unendurable, bringing me to my outermost limits, where life and death are one and the same.

I could never have imagined the existence of such a powerful force; and yet, this force is nothing more than life itself.

The singing—rather, the conscious screaming, or even better the breathing, the loud toning exhalation—helped me to keep from getting lost in the storm, which was blustering unrestrainedly like a raging fury.

The tone stopped me from going under and drowning. Through it I sensed and understood: I could expect or desire support from no one except myself. Nothing and nobody from outside could help me. The tone forced me to concentrate continually upon myself, my inner I. It forced me into an absolute here and now. And so, amidst this churning ocean, I did not capsize and was out of danger.

The delivery stage went much more quickly, with an incomparable, liberating feeling of exaltation at every contraction.

Finally, the almost magical moment came: the child was out. I opened my eyes and saw my husband crying with joy. He said: "My darling, Martino is born. You've done it." Yes, I'd done it. I'd managed, all alone, without an episiotomy, to bring this baby into the world.

And so we two, this new creature and I, looked each other directly in the eye. I was still in a trance, somewhat battered, and full of bliss at this new being, this wrinkly and slightly gray-faced child, who was so quiet, not at all disoriented, and not crying either. *O* and *A* tones came from his mouth. And then Martino began to sing. . . .

My husband and I laughed out loud, drunk on happiness.

I had become a mother.

A look, a smile from this child, and I bubbled over with endless gratitude for this life that had been given to me.

Martino is now three and a half months old. When I think of my giving birth I am filled with joy, and I am proud to have experienced that birth so intensively and so successfully.

Again, many thanks for everything I learned from you in your seminar.

❧ *Commentary*

First, many thanks for this beautiful letter and for such a brilliant analysis of each individual step, showing how enormously important it is to concentrate. The moment your attention is no longer directed to the here and now, the moment you lose yourself in your thoughts, the moment you stop being a witness as you so wonderfully express it—in that brief disconnection, that instant in which you think of something else—you will become a victim, prey to terrible pains, a wreck close to sinking.

And this pure energy of the tone will fetch you back into the here and now.

1. Why did you lie down in bed as soon as you entered the clinic? A bed is for sick people, not for giving birth. But in the clinic, it's all they know. You get sent to bed, and as soon as you're in the bed, you play your role: you're in pain, you're sick.

   I repeat: bringing a child into the world is a joy, and not an illness. For this reason: Don't ever lie down in bed! Walk up and down, pace back and forth, without shoes, of course, and without slippers or socks. As I said before, all the acupuncture meridians start from your feet, which act as an aid to your perceptions. And you should walk slowly, attentively, scrupulously, accompanying every step with a long exhalation.

2. On all fours in bed? Why? That's not advisable.

3. Keeping your eyes closed? Here again, why? You know the old saying: where the hand goes the eyes go, where the eyes go the hand goes. So keep your eyes open and keep looking at your hand!

4. Your partner's hand in yours? No! Do you need your mother when you're lying in your lover's arms? The first time, perhaps, you were a *little* anxious. But you didn't shout out "Help! Mom!" did you?

   You said that in these moments of feeling completely beside yourself, you learned and understood once and for all that you could expect no help from anyone else, that you alone could help yourself, and that you could count only on yourself. Wasn't that the most important lesson you learned?

   And the tone saved you, directed you toward your own center and toward what was going on in you. This and only this saved you on the spot and prevented you from going under and drowning.

5. When your child was finally born, when he came out of you, you opened your eyes. And the first person you looked at was . . . your husband.

   No! This first gaze must go to the child, who—even if you disbelieve this—can only feel betrayed otherwise. Don't you know that you can't simultaneously turn your attention to multiple people, but only to one person, because in doing so you have to look at the person? It is impossible for you to look at your husband and child at the same time. And who has the first claim? The baby! Isn't that obvious?

Anyway, in the next instant you looked directly into your child's eyes. In this moment your husband no longer existed. And there was only the child and you.

"You haven't thrown me out the door, have you? Do you love me, then? Do you still love me?" That is the great question that you see and recognize in the eyes of this child. The answer he so anxiously expects from you is: "But of course I love you! That's why I wanted to give you your freedom!" And so the child's fundamental fear of having lost your love is dispelled.

But with this question, "Do you love me?" there is also: "Do you really love me, only me, and no one else? Because if you love me, if you really love me, you can love only me and no one else." If the father is present, for the child he represents the Other. How can the child then feel that he/she alone is loved, that there is no other?

The whole drama surrounding the birth that is common practice today, with the whole family crowding around the newborn, is absolutely absurd.

6. I assume that someone gave you an injection as soon as you arrived in the clinic, which hindered you from walking. And I am sure that someone gave you oxytocin to activate the contractions. This is why your dilation stage went so quickly and why there was no breathing pause between the contractions, which were

"subintrant." This is the term used when one contraction directly follows another, without any interruption. This makes the labor agonizing.

How brave you must have been not to ask for, or indeed demand, peridural anesthesia as so many other women do. With so much courage, all I can do is express my admiration. And I am simply astonished that the tone itself was so effective in such a "pathological" situation.

You will surely have learned from this that you should have your next child in a place where you are completely safe—safe, that is, from any medical manipulation.

Sabine L., Verdabbio, Switzerland

First letter

Dear Mr. Leboyer,

My youngest son Lüzza was born at home on February 25, shortly after I attended your seminar in Bellinzona.

The birth was quite simply wonderful. With the first contraction I started singing. The sound of the tambūrā on the cassette *Breathing and Singing* accompanied me.*

For me, it was like the trapeze artist's net, giving me a feeling of security.

The whole time, I paid attention to my body's posture and made sure to sit as correctly as possible, moving gently forward and backward to the tones, especially the vowels *E* and *I.*

During the pauses between the contractions that always came just as I expected them to, I was able to fully enjoy the calm.

But what was most surprising to me was something that in fact seemed almost unbelievable: the stronger the labor pains became, the stronger my voice gave out the tones. My voice did not become weaker, but ever stronger. I also had the impression that this voice, reaching right to my belly, was changing itself into a great energy.

From time to time my voice rose up high, then I lost

---

*The harmonic tone of the tambūrā should accompany the woman when she is passing through contractions and birth as if through a terrific storm. Its purpose is to keep her safe from "shipwreck" and to make the journey into a wonderful "crossing" instead.

control. But Iris, my midwife, who had also attended the seminar, helped me to find the right tone again, bringing everything back into equilibrium. Other than this, she never intervened. She was simply there with me, as a silent observer.

I had given birth before, but never in such a clear state of consciousness. This time, thanks to the singing, I followed my child. I accompanied him. I felt how he was pushing his way outward, toward the light.

I can truly say that right to the end, I remained the "captain of my ship." I didn't let myself go off course for a single instant. And even at the end, during the delivery stage, I accompanied every contraction with a tone. I felt this tone like an arrow pointing out the direction in which I had to press.

Finally my son was born, and what a marvel, he came into the world without a cry. I lay on my back right away, since in labor I had instinctively gone on all fours. Iris placed my child on my belly—an indescribable, unforgettable moment.

Never before had I been filled with such joy.

❧ *Commentary*

Sabine wrote in her letter: "the stronger the labor pains became . . ." and so I asked her in what sense she used the term "labor pains." Didn't she rather mean "contractions," which have for so long been incorrectly called "pains"?

I wanted to know whether it actually went badly for

her, whether she suffered. Or did she just mean that these contractions kept getting stronger?

Her answer was clear: "You are right, Mr. Leboyer, when I wrote about labor pains I actually meant the contractions that were longer and stronger each time. You are right, I didn't choose the right word. It didn't go badly for me for a single moment, and I didn't suffer. On the contrary, I was fulfilled, overcome by an indescribable feeling of peace and harmony. In everything I experienced there was no room for suffering or fear."

Second letter

Dear Mr. Leboyer,

October 13 is an important date for me, because my husband and I met each other twenty years ago on this day. It is a day that invites me to look back.

If I were to tally things up, I could say that the birth of my youngest son Lüzza was the most beautiful moment of my life. I often think of it and am touched again and again.

This kind of birth, in joy and harmony, has very strongly influenced my relationship to Lüzza. I have a patience with him that I have never mustered before in my life.

I am glad you are writing a book on "The Art of Giving Birth." It will be a great help for those women who have the courage and wisdom to follow this path.

After giving birth, I have often discussed it with other women, or at least wanted to, and I keep trying. But I have found that in general they are very afraid and would rather not hear anything about it. And women who had a more or less decent birth behind them didn't want to know anything about how a woman can give birth joyfully. They didn't believe it, they were even mistrusting, and they had plenty of good excuses for not wanting to hear about it. I had to admit that I wasn't able to persuade them.

I hope your book will help women to accept their fear but not to be dominated by it.

You once said that one must look directly into the eyes of fear like a samurai, and make fear itself afraid. I am very fond of this image.

At the moment when I was truly afraid, it suddenly seemed to me as if the fear was afraid. And so I was freed from it.

How can I thank you? Thank you for giving me the greatest joy of my life!

Luciana B., Parma

My name is Luciana.

I was fortunate to attend your seminar here in Parma shortly before the birth of my second child.

The first time I gave birth, I had cervical tearing, which caused postpartum bleeding, which is no joke. I barely avoided having to have a caesarian section.

In my current situation, what I learned in the seminar—the movements, singing, and answers to my questions—led to much reflection. I realized, I understood, that there is another way of giving birth, and that I had only gone into the hospital because I had, in fact, imagined that someone other than myself was going to bring my child into the world.

This time, quite calmly, I made a new decision: my child would be born at home.

Since I needed some support for my decision, I told the Home Birth Association about my decision. After they heard me out, discussed it, and talked things over with me, their answer was unfortunately in the negative. After everything that happened with the birth of my first child, I was decisively advised against a home birth. This made me very angry.

I was ready to face this great monster of fear with my head held high. I would not let myself be ordered around any longer. I, and no other, would bring little Anita into the world. Especially since this time I no longer felt lost but was ready to support myself with the song that I had learned and that had filled me.

On the morning of June 30, the contractions began, at first quite light, regular, and already rhythmical. What a difference from my first birth, at which the contractions were violent and completely uncontrolled, tearing me apart in the most literal sense of the word.

On the contrary, I enjoyed my contractions this time and felt that my little Anita would come to me thanks to these contractions. As things progressed, the contractions soon became much stronger. But right at the beginning, I had begun to sing, and I kept it up all the way through this very long, magnificent experience.

I stayed at home throughout the dilation phase. I only went to the hospital once I was having extremely strong contractions. (Why didn't I just stay at home?) I never stopped singing. I sang in the car and kept singing as I walked into the hospital. I sang so loud they told me they couldn't hear the baby's heartbeat any longer. (In fact, their equipment wasn't working properly.) I kept singing when they told me they couldn't position the baby's head properly. I could feel the baby pressing hard on my perineum. When they asked me if they could pop the amniotic sac, I answered: No!

I kept singing and massaged the two shiatsu points, and the amniotic fluid spilled out. I pressed four times, and Anita was there. She had made the jump into life, as happy as a colt, as if she wanted to say: "Hello, here I am, I've arrived!"

Everything went so pleasantly. How different, what a

contrast to my first birth! I missed out on so many things in the clinic when I believed others were going to fetch my baby into the world. And what would have happened to me if I had once again gone into the hospital right at the beginning?

I want to tell you that this child has changed everything in my life, and I cannot thank you enough.

❧ *Commentary*

Does this even need any commentary?

This is another very revealing example, showing what women believe and what they continue to be led to believe: that they cannot give birth alone, that they need someone to fetch their child for them, to pull it out of them.

What can I say about the negative advice from the Home Birth Association, which was only dictated by fear?

Sara A., Parma

Dear Mr. Leboyer,

My name is Sara.

I was fortunate enough to attend your seminar in Parma in May. I was at the end of my pregnancy, and thanks to tai chi lessons and Kanarese singing to the sound of the tambūrā, I became aware of how important posture and breathing are.

And so I would like to give you my immeasurable thanks, because after everything I learned, discovered, and understood from you, my childbirth experience was simply wonderful.

I gave birth at home. It was nighttime and only my midwife and husband were with me, in total quiet.

During the whole dilation phase I walked, swaying back and forth, up and down. Above all other things I was completely concentrated on what was going on inside me. The breathing I had learned (never from the chest, always from the abdomen) was very helpful to me.

There were so many small details to attend to: inclining my head forward so that all tension would leave my neck, keeping my shoulders down, and the whole time taking care to breathe as slowly as possible. To breathe? No, I mean to breathe out.

Breathing out became slower all by itself in the course of labor, with the increasingly stronger and more powerful contractions.

Very often, while walking around in the rest periods, I repeated "Yes, Lord! Yes, Lord!" and leaned forward, relaxing

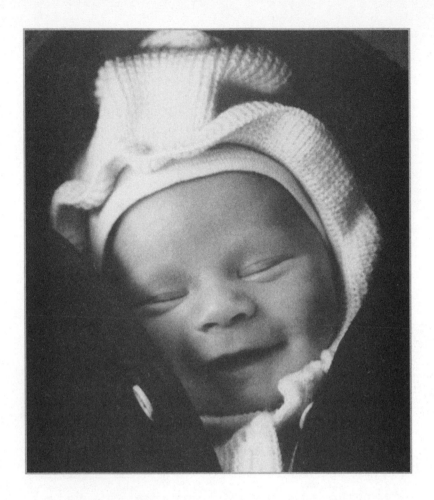

my back. At the same time I turned ever more deeply inward, and with my whole heart took in what was happening inside me, what was coming to pass.

At some point the amniotic sac burst and I had time to drop to the floor and go on all fours. After two contractions, Lorenzo was lying in my arms.

What really astounded me was the fact that this time I could feel each contraction coming and was able to accompany it with my breathing. When my first child was born, the contractions were simply awful, terrifying, uncontrollable. This time, unbelievably, I could accompany the contractions with my breathing until they subsided, and so, astonishingly, grasp what they were accomplishing. As improbable as it may seem, I actually did not suffer at all this time.

How can I thank you, and how can I explain to you that this birth was the most beautiful thing I have ever experienced?

Stefanie S., Freiburg im Breisgau

Dear Frédérick,

After I learned from you about the tai chi chuan movements and toning to the sound of the tambūrā, I prepared other women and accompanied them during their births. Every time I became more and more persuaded that this was the right way.

Now I have had a child of my own. I myself was able to have this magnificent, fantastic adventure that is bringing a child into the world.

The tambūrā and the movements both accompanied me the whole time.

How can I ever thank you enough?

I must agree with you: yes, it is true, it is possible to remain captain on board one's ship amidst this storm, this tornado, and to not go under, not get shipwrecked in the hurricane of childbirth.

Eugenia C., Parma

Dear Mr. Leboyer,

Our daughter Gemma came into the world in the morning's gentle light and barely perceptible wind. She was born with the tone and from the tone. Thanks to this tone she has seen the light of the world.

Ah, what strength and what grandeur the *A* has!* It seemed as if it would break through the earth like a volcano. The radiant *E* connected the earth with the concentrated energy of the water, leaving it supple and open. The *I* filled me with a crystal clear energy and taught me of all the beauty and greatness of this gift. The *O* let me tumble enchanted into the exquisite perfection of the universe. The *U* brought me to a humble obeisance before the immeasurable vastness of the universe. The *M* finally allowed me to see the divine in life. The labor, like the late stage of pregnancy, was like a marvelous, wonderful journey of unspeakable power. The tone made my body vibrate and made me conscious of what it means to exist; it brought me with ease into harmony, a harmony that was no longer my own and that, thankfully, I could not resist. Gemma was born at home. Through the open window the last glow of the vanishing summer shone upon us.

How can I thank you for what you have taught us and revealed to us!

---

*The singing of the tones *A, E, O, I, U, M* to the tambūrā will be explained in part 2 of this book.

Delphine A., Crest, France

Dear Frédérick Leboyer,

Six months ago today, "My Lord" was born.

I need to describe to you in simple words how I experienced this birth. Simple but true words, which reflect what I learned on each of the weekend seminars with you.

I think that what helped me most in giving birth was the image of being a captain at the rudder of a ship.

I still remember one of the films, *Waves of Life*, the waves, toning to the sound of the tambūrā, and I remember the sound of the roaring water, becoming louder and louder. Even then I could feel how much this touched me, how deeply it reached me.

As I was giving birth to Stéphane, I again had the feeling I experienced while I was in the seminar, doing the exercises, and watching the films, bringing to mind this simple phrase: even in the strongest storm, the captain still steers her ship.

My impression is that this phrase gave me the strength to master the waves (the contractions), even as they grew stronger and stronger. I was sure that the storm would let up eventually. Also, I could let this tone out of myself as loudly as I wanted to. I had a feeling of being centered—yes, that's the right word, centered—and oriented around my midpoint.

And something else peculiar happened: Although I noticed everything that was going on around me during this time, and heard everything that was said, at the same time there was a great distance between me and the outside world, as if I was absent, just focused on myself and my baby. I was absolutely in my center.

In fact, I already knew about this very specific feeling from when we practiced the series of movements over and over in the seminar. I felt like I was entirely directed toward the center, and the movements allowed me to sense every cell of my body. This was so good.

So there it is. I just wanted to thank you for having been my guide in the discovery of my inner strength, my womanly power.

Yes, I simply want to thank you.

❧ *Commentary*

"My Lord," as Delphine calls her child at the beginning of this letter, is an allusion to the gentle movement of the head, which is inclined forward during the exercises. This releases tension in the neck, which is the starting point of all tension in the body. This slightly inclined head also signifies a "yes." It is a sign of acceptance and submission. It indicates a greeting, a reverence expressing respect shown to another, for example a person of rank, a prince.

This greeting is, in a sense, hidden and is only perceptible to those who have a special perceptiveness for it.

"Yes, My Lord!" also evokes the statement: "Let your will be done!"

Is this Lord a god, a demiurge? Not in the least. This Lord, to whose will the woman can only conform, is very simply the child in her. This child is the true helmsman on the dangerous voyage through the storm of birth. And as the saying goes, the child is the father of mankind. This is the most important message of *Birth without Violence*: as you are received, so you will be.

"Yes!" This is not meant symbolically, but entirely prosaically. It is the opposite of the lamentable "iron fist." Don't resist, but accept! Do not meet force with equal and opposite force, with the aggressiveness of an opponent. No! Otherwise your power will fall into the void!

"Yes, My Lord!"

Beatrice B., Bologna

Dear Mr. Leboyer,

My name is Beatrice.

I live in Bologna, where I teach yoga primarily to pregnant women.

At this time I would like to thank you for teaching me about the art of Kanarese singing,* which I used during my two pregnancies and which allowed me to experience giving birth both times in a truly remarkable way. It made me able to become conscious of the sacred character of this event and to marvel at the astonishing and unbelievably strong power that built up within me from contraction to contraction, and how precisely and skillfully I was able to regulate them. Not to mention the deep, intense, indescribably intelligent look that newborn children have when they have been given the time to see the light of the world in their own rhythm, without rushing things.

---

*Kanarese singing originates in southern India. In part 2 of this book, and on the CD, a simplified version of this singing is presented.

INDUCED LABOR

Silvia P., Pavia

The following letter was written by a woman who first did yoga exercises during her pregnancy, then discovered the tai chi movements and toning to the sound of the tambūrā at a seminar in Monte-Isola.

Unfortunately, when her water broke, contractions didn't begin. This often happens, and the woman should not worry about it. It can simply be a fissure in the amniotic sac, some small tears, or a secondary rupture in the sac. She should stay at home and measure her body temperature; as long as she doesn't have a fever, there is no reason for concern. She can wait for several days without worry.

In clinics, where people live in constant fear of being legally prosecuted and having to go through a lawsuit, they regrettably decide to induce labor instead of patiently waiting. They love to step in and take over the "rudder." But this never leads to good results, because every child must be born at its proper time.

This woman apparently had a premonition of what would happen to her. She writes:

"My pregnancy was easy and relaxed. I wasn't afraid of pain, but was certainly scared of medical intervention."

And that's exactly what happened to her. The contractions didn't set in, so they raised the oxytocin dose in her injections—resulting in contractions. But the contractions were horribly, unbearably strong.

Because of the IV, they chained her to the bed, so she could not walk as she had learned to do and would have gladly done. But she sat up in bed, being careful to keep a good posture, and began to sing. How extraordinarily brave!

Since her cervix didn't open, and she couldn't bear it any longer—the contractions had gone on for a long time—she asked, ashamed though she was, for peridural anesthesia. After the shot, the "monster," the hellish pain, was gone. Half an hour later it was all over; her child was born. At least induced labor saved her from the customary caesarian section.

In another letter she writes:

The brutal contractions were beyond anything one can imagine. When I think back on giving birth, my memory is of suffering terribly, and of failing. (The pains were simply due to the injection and to the whole completely unnatural process.) Despite everything, singing was my companion in need, it was the Ariadne's thread, leading me along, giving me a feeling of irrepressible strength and even of joy. When I think back on the birth, it seems like an initiation ritual to me. Everything played out despite my own will. In a certain sense, it was like dying, to be reborn on another level.

It is inexplicable—as if the woman herself is being reborn. It's as if, during this terrific experience, one is sensing love, a universal love, embracing everything that lives in creation.

G's children, Greece

These are photos of two children, born to the same mother, who came into the world in entirely different ways. For the first child, C, contractions were induced artificially (we won't go into the reasons for this here). As is always the case with induced labor, the contractions were very intense. The mother endured this very bravely, without asking for peridural anesthesia.

The effects of this "violence" are clearly visible in the facial expression of the baby, both at the time of birth and much later. Above all, this violence caused the girl to develop a specific personality: she is a very anxious child who often appears fearful and worried.

With the second child, however, the contractions came on entirely spontaneously, and the mother was fully aware of the significance of breathing during labor. And so this girl developed a completely different personality, both at the time of birth and years later, throughout her life: she is a truly "radiant" child, not only full of joy but also so talented that she is expected to be a great musician when she grows up.

Scientifically speaking, there is something remarkable here: for a long time, it was commonly believed that our personalities depend on genes alone. Here is the proof that this is not true! Our personalities are tremendously dependent on the mother's condition during pregnancy, on conditions during labor and birth, and on how the child is received upon its arrival into the world!

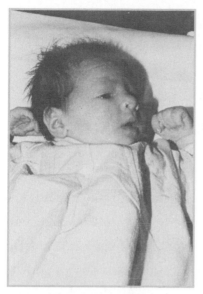
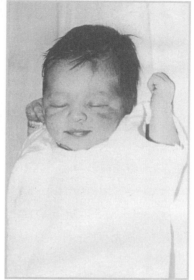
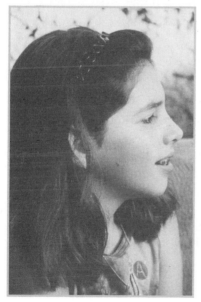
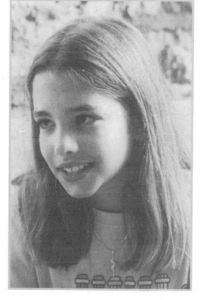

C
FIRST CHILD
INDUCED LABOR

M
SECOND CHILD
NATURAL BIRTH
CORRECT BREATHING BY THE
MOTHER DURING CONTRACTIONS

CAESARIAN SECTION

Beatrix K., Budapest

Dear Frédérick,

Thank you for your interest in the story of my last birth, on which I myself think back so often. Honestly, I talk about it all the time, without anyone listening to me, I'm afraid.

It has gradually become clear to me that only a few people—a few women—are in a position to understand me. Those who had a caesarian section like I did, and who are now expecting another child, don't say: "So is it true? It's possible to give birth in the normal way?" Sadly, they don't ask that. Instead of listening to me and marveling at what I have done, they think I'm crazy, a woman with no idea of responsibility, playing with her own life and the life of her child. They believe I was lucky to survive the whole thing in the first place.

My pregnancy was problem-free. Apart from a few minor problems at the beginning, I can truly say that I felt happy and calm the whole time. And I was lucky enough to find a midwife, the only one in Hungary, who undertook to deliver me—or I mean, to accompany me through giving birth. Despite the two caesarian sections I have had previously, she declared that it was a good decision for me to give birth normally this time.

After my decision was made, I prepared myself. Of course I had the initial examinations, but later I felt not the slightest desire to have these monthly checks into which women are forced these days.

I visited my midwife from time to time. Over coffee

in her kitchen, I could discuss with her the questions that occurred to me—the things that moved my heart.

Thankfully, I didn't listen to all the horror stories people kept telling me about such and such a catastrophic birth. . . .

I also didn't listen to well-meaning advice: What, you're not having amniocentesis? And you're not having an ultrasound every month?

I only read books that talked about what a marvel a birth is.

In spite of this, I had to find a clinic for the birth. For each of my first two births, my caesarian sections, I went into an unknown clinic, into "no man's land." It was terrible being surrounded by entirely unknown and apathetic people.

Agnes took me to a professor who did an ultrasound to assess the scar on my uterus. When he saw that the scar was only 6 mm wide, he said: "Madam, with such a thin and delicate scar, there is no question of a natural birth. Your scar could break at the first contraction, and burst your uterus. Your child could die! And we would have to do an emergency operation and remove the uterus."

His emphatic decree was: "Caesarian section by appointment, at least a week before the projected birth date. Then we will remove your child."

You can't imagine how disappointed I was or how much fear he caused me.

The whole family, including my husband, who is a pediatrician, was glad someone had given me a talking-to. My own sister said to me: "I hope you will finally stop reading these ridiculous books about the beauty of birth. When there's a risk, and here there is definitely a risk, then you can only choose the safe way."

Fortunately, Agnes was of a different opinion. The 6 mm scar didn't impress her at all. She simply wanted to find another clinic. But first she visited the professor again. He told her adamantly: "I have made it a rule for myself: after a caesarian section, especially after two, there is no question of a natural birth. For your friend, this means a caesarian section prior to the predicted date of birth. If she won't listen to me, she can go to the devil!"

For a day after that I was very upset. But Agnes said she would find another hospital next morning.

Luckily, my water broke that same night. I say "luckily" because this moment was a turning point: as if by a miracle, it all became entirely clear in my mind. The questions I had so often asked myself vanished. Instead, I felt a great calm. No frightening ideas were able to wreck my composure now.

I called Agnes up, and she told me to lie back down again.

"Impossible," I responded. I was too excited. I asked her to come to me. I didn't want to be alone. My husband hadn't even woken up the whole time.

Agnes came, and she examined me. My cervix was now open 5 cm. I took a nice warm bath—it was winter and I felt a bit cold. Then I called up a close friend who had given birth to four of her own children with Agnes attending. With the two of them at my side, I felt completely safe.

And from this moment on, it was as if a miracle was occurring. There was only one worry for me: finding the right position so that everything could take its course. I felt as if I was on another planet. Time had ceased to exist. What I remember is my voice, and how I applied what I learned from you. I wasn't conscious of the fact that I tried to bring my contractions and the tones into harmony. It happened spontaneously, all by itself.

How long did all this go on? I have no idea. The contractions lasted about eight hours, but I wouldn't have been able to say whether it was an hour or a year.

Did I suffer? Oh, no. It was strange, but I never had a long moment of pain. I could even say that my contractions, the waves, were quite gentle, better than bearable. Only the delivery was harder. Perhaps the contractions weren't strong enough. Agnes encouraged me to press harder as the contractions stopped. The child's head began to poke out. I could touch him. What an experience! But then he went back in again. During this last stage, my voice was what saved me. It was so wonderful, letting it out of myself without the least inhibition. Any attempt to control me was doomed to failure.

Finally, Fabian was born and was laid in my arms.

Unfortunately, I began to bleed at this moment. The placenta did not come loose. Agnes didn't think she was a match for this, especially because I'd had two caesarians, and so we drove to the hospital. There they gave me total anesthesia so they could take the placenta out and assess the condition of my womb. It was intact. The scar (6 mm) had not broken.

A final word about my husband: As I mentioned earlier, he was still sleeping when my contractions set in. But finally we woke him up to ask his advice. Should we go to the clinic? He answered that he had . . . no opinion! And so, thank heaven, I gave birth at home, and did it perfectly, despite my two caesarians.

I hope my example will give courage to women who find themselves in the same situation. Because now I can say: I'd had two children, but I didn't know what it really meant to *have* a child. Now I truly know what it means to become a mother.

❧ Commentary

The professor who ordered a third caesarian section by reason of the potentially dangerous uterine scar was correct—from his scientific, logical point of view. But Beatrix, with her knowledge as a woman—and as a woman expecting a child—was also right. Has science not taught us that logic and intellect cannot be held accountable when it comes down to reality? As for the rules on which the professor based his decision, they show that he, with his rigid position, was in the wrong.

The midwife advised Beatrix to lie down again after the amniotic sac burst. But that was a mistake. She had forgotten, or did not know, that the woman must walk back and forth once contractions have begun. In doing this, as we have mentioned before, she must pay attention to each of her steps, put each foot down starting with the heel, and accompany each step with her breathing.

Driving her to the clinic during the hemorrhaging—that

is, the bleeding following the birth—was another mistake. Stimulating discharge of the placenta is not a problem; it must be done immediately. But during the ride to the hospital, the bleeding could have become life threatening. Perhaps midwives in Hungary do not know this.

What to say about the husband who kept on sleeping, and who, when he was awakened and asked what to do, answered: "I don't know, I have no opinion"? Quite simply: he was right. Only women truly know themselves. Childbirth is their secret garden.

❧ *Conclusion:*
Arguments against Caesarian Section

Caesarian section, often touted as the safest method in modern times, should certainly not be banned; but it should only be performed in "high risk" cases. There are two reasons for this:

The first reason relates to the child, who (unconsciously) has the feeling (and will retain this feeling throughout life): "Aha! I've done it! I came out into the world thanks to my own strength! Yes, I did it, I escaped from the cave, from the prison. If I hadn't been able to get out, I would have suffocated, died, been crushed." (Think of Plato's cave allegory!) But with a caesarian section, the child needs outside help to save itself and to be saved, leading to a perpetually "dependent" life, always surrendering to the will of others. Such a person will never be autonomous.

The second argument against caesarian section is the

necessity for anesthesia, even if it is so highly developed. It should be avoided at all costs. Why? Because it separates mother and child from one another during the moment when their mutual exertion is absolutely necessary for life. Birth is an adventure experienced by both. Mother and child must remain in contact the whole time; otherwise the child will feel betrayed. It will feel deserted by its mother when its life is in the greatest danger. *De profundis clamavi!* (Out of the depths I cry to you!)

Anesthesia requires inevitable separation. It numbs the woman and her perceptions (to a greater or lesser extent) but has no effect at all upon the child's perceptions. And so the two, who should be as one, are like strangers. The inner connection, the "bonding" between mother and child, the feeling of belonging together, breaks in two. The woman "has" a child instead of becoming a mother.

A certain animal breeder named Marais once wondered why his goats and sheep should have to suffer while giving birth. He was sure animals suffered when delivering their young (which is strenuous for them, but strain doesn't mean suffering), and so he gave them chloroform or ether. The result was that the animals did not recognize their young. They turned away from them and refused to suckle them. The experiment was repeated with peridural anesthesia and yielded the same result—for the same reason. And the same is true for humans. Here is a convincing example:

Some time ago, I received a letter from a woman who told me she had tried desperately to make contact with me because I had brought her into the world when I was still working as an obstetrician. Naturally, I invited the woman to visit me, and she told me her story.

She was French, born in Paris, and lived in Switzerland. She was qualified as a midwife but had not yet conducted a birth. Her life seemed like total martyrdom: ten years of psychoanalysis, and then ten years of craniosacral therapy, both as a patient and to get a diploma so that she could practice in this field. Because instead of guiding women through giving birth, she only prepared them for it.

How had she herself been born? She wanted to know whether I had anesthetized her mother during the birth. Yes, her mother had been sedated.

And the result reminded me of Marais's experiment with his sheep and goats: the mother did not breastfeed the baby after she woke up from her anesthesia. And even worse, she did not raise the child but entrusted it to the care of the grandparents.

Because her mother had never cared for her—even though she had been raised lovingly by her grandparents—this young woman had been an emotional "cripple" throughout her life. And so she went in search of the reason, just as one might search for some fatal trauma by going through psychoanalysis.

Mea culpa? At the time, neither I nor anyone else knew how greatly the effects of anesthesia during birth could damage an entire life. I only learned it near the end of my professional years. And I will venture to say—although it requires a great deal of courage and honesty—that I changed my method of delivery from the ground up. I was brave enough to give up, once and for all, administering the anesthesia that I used to give liberally to all the women, and for which reason they had trusted in me so much, leading me to become rich and famous.

Letter from Dr. Hans Neumann, Obstetrician from Leonding, Austria

Today there are an increasing number of obstetricians who are not worthy of the title. When a woman wants a caesarian, they say: It is her right. But most of these doctors do not act in the interest of the woman or child; rather they act to reduce their own fear. Others base their decisions on convenience, and many are motivated simply by financial reasons.

Luckily, there are still doctors of the old school, who are horrified by what is done to women and children in our so-called developed nations, allegedly for reasons of safety.

Increasingly medicalized and mechanized obstetrics does not increase safety but only intensifies the fear that leads women to want caesarian sections to assuage this fear—which we have produced.

How ashamed our practitioners should be! How many caesarian sections are performed without true safety reasons?!

What bloody splendid medicine!

There is a story about a woman (proudly) saying that thanks to peridural anesthesia, she watched television while giving birth. Another was able to finish her crossword puzzle. A third, who chose to have a scheduled caesarian, said: "I checked in!" (as if she'd reserved a room at a hotel). "I just had to register, and from that point on I didn't have to worry about a thing! Why should I go through all that fear and anxiety, all that pain, when it can all be done without me having to participate? Everything was organized ahead of time, and it was really wonderful!"

All these things took place in the United States. We Europeans can do nothing better than follow their example. After all, isn't the United States at the forefront of modern medicine?

℘

The following promises are made by a clinic whose name I will not give. I will not even mention what country this clinic is in. What is offered here is standard everywhere.

COME TO US TO GIVE BIRTH!
We are at your disposal, and we promise
that your birth will be:
On time
Quick
Gentle
Painless
Safe
Home-like
Caesarian section on request!

It sounds like a dream—or rather, a nightmare.

What more can one add, except that it is incomprehensible?

Peridural anesthesia is something sensational in all these so-called modern, well-equipped hospitals. It is performed on order, and people do not see the damage that can result from it. The anesthetists themselves are not even aware of it.

What damage can occur?

Peridural anesthesia separates the mother from the child. The necessary contact, so important for life, is interrupted.

Furthermore, the birth loses its deeper meaning. It is meant to be like a "rite of passage," an initiation ritual, a lesson of courage and patience, something we all need badly in life. What makes a successful birth? The joy we experience together? No—the trials we overcome together.

In the course of giving birth, something in the woman dies and is reborn. "A maiden dies and is reborn as a mother."

It is the difference between *having* and *being*.

With peridural anesthesia, the woman just has a child. When she gives birth consciously, she finally becomes a mother, and finally truly a woman.

THE MIRACLE OF BIRTH

I do not wish to conclude this chapter with stories that give us reason for dishonor and shame.

Here then are a couple of other letters on the miracle of birth.

Letter from an Older Woman, Canada

All that is needed, all that is wanted at the time of birth is to be very quiet and on one's own.

Yes, at this point you want to be by yourself because anything coming from the world outside truly intrudes.

You have become so acutely sensitive that the slightest false note is like a stab. An unwanted question, people moving around, carelessly even a noise, a door banging grates at your ears, hurts—and the magic is gone.

Fear?

Oh, no! You feel you're protected as if standing in a magic circle where nothing can touch you.

You are under the protection, the blessings of infinite Light and Love embodied in your child.

Yes, you are under the protection of this little one on its way to you.

Marie G., Athens

Dear Mr. Leboyer,

Every time I immerse myself in your book *Das Fest der Geburt* [A Celebration of Birth]* with the view of the newborn it presents, I once again experience this great adventure of birth, which is now quite some time in the past.

I feel the fear and the joy. I look death right in the face. I try to experience everything consciously, to keep my eyes open and at the same time to direct my view inward. I flow with the waves and lose myself in them. I am ready, I open myself, I fall into ecstasy, and then, finally free, I let myself loose into eternity.

Everything is calm, and I sense how the ego disappears; I savor the outpouring of perception, the tenderness and fullness of the child in me.

You wrote: "As if life could be nourished by calculation! As if poetry could flourish without love!" These words moved me to tears, without my knowing why. But I wanted to thank you for this.

---

*Frédérick Leboyer, *Das Fest der Geburt* (Munich: Kösel, 1982). Out of print.

Sarah B., St. Paulin, Canada

Thank you again for this tenderness, this building of courage, these images of life.

During the two times I gave birth, I felt I was hearing your voice, even though I don't know it. It was speaking of a ship, a storm, a captain, and waves. Your words drew me out of the labor pains, out of the fear into which I was in danger of falling, of drowning. The sentences came out from my innermost depths.

You know, I believe the babies understand you when we read to them from your book. They go with us into secret places and take hold of the most subtle and wonderful things that exist in life. My children are now five and seven years old.

Even today, sometimes I still silently thank you. I still leaf through your books and show them to people. They remain my first reference. Your work is so big-hearted, full of empathy, and it does so much endless good

You have given me, my children, and many other people a pure and simple life, a clear and strong message, a powerful support, and above all, such a deep understanding.

Thank you.

May all the love that you have shared fulfill you, and may peace be with you.

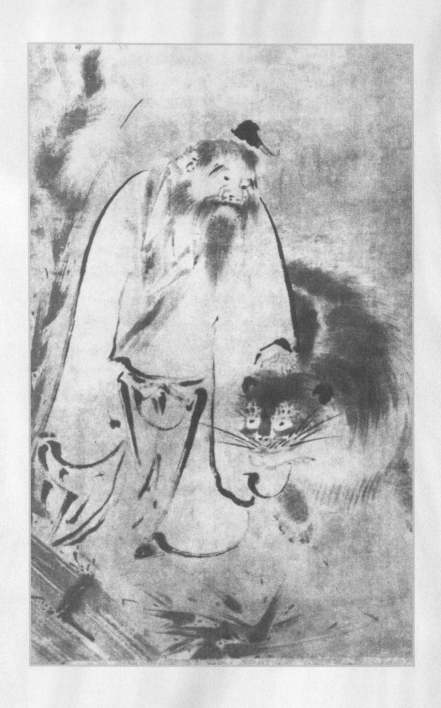

PART TWO

The Art of Breathing and Singing

Breathing

Dear Lisa,

Now we must part. But not before we are standing with both feet on the ground.

And this means: Not before I have spoken with you about breathing, which plays a crucial role. Only breathing can save you in the progress of this great adventure, in your crossing through this great storm. The breathing that naturally also causes so much confusion on your end, that is so poorly taught—this breathing alone can save you, or in the opposite case, when it is not taught to you correctly, can be cataclysmic for you.

Giving birth is like weathering a storm. The only thing that protects the woman from shipwreck, that can stop her boat from going under and sinking, the only thing that truly helps her to arrive at the harbor safe and sound, even smiling and radiating joy—with her precious cargo—is her breathing. Or to be specific, her breath, and how long it lasts!

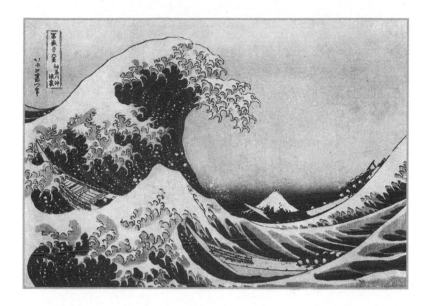

Nowadays, this is no longer a secret to anyone. But what kind of breathing is it?

Lamentably, the breathing techniques taught to pregnant women in numerous preparation courses for so-called painless birth are of no more value than the other information with which they are bombarded. This includes a horde of complications that can arise during childbirth, but without mentioning how rare these are—naturally only increasing women's fear.

Let us look at some of the breathing techniques that are taught and are of absolutely no use to women:

1. The so-called small dog breathing, a gasping and superficial breathing method originating from yoga, in which it is called *bhastrika,* meaning bellows, and is used for replenishing energy. This breathing can only

be useful to the woman right at the end of the birth, when she may press too strongly and risk tearing.

This is a type of breathing that should only be practiced for a short amount of time, and is absolutely not appropriate for the longest and most strenuous— not to mention the most painful—stage of birth, i.e., cervical dilation.

2. "Breathe in, hold your breath"—another breathing technique that should only be applied at the end of labor, when the woman is beginning to squeeze.

"Breathe in! Take a deep breathe! And now squeeze!"

This breathing—inhaling, holding your breath, pressing—also comes from yoga, but its only result is that the poor woman's face grows red, then purple, her eyes become bloodshot, and she gets terribly dizzy. This breathing technique is absolutely not advisable!

In addition, the two aforementioned breathing techniques involve chest breathing, which one should simply give up and which is only ever advisable during the end stage of birth, the delivery stage.

What sorts of breathing, then, are advised for the longest and most painful stage of cervical dilation?

3. So-called circular breathing, continuously breathing in and out in the upper chest area, is absolutely to be avoided. Breathing in and out without interruption is the exact opposite of what a woman giving birth should do. It is a type of breathing common in

"rebirthing," a breathing technique that can bring to the surface feelings buried in the subconscious that are associated with the woman's own birth. Reliving negative feelings in this way will lead the woman to fall back into anxiety, and her ship will run aground.

What can we conclude from all this? How should the woman breathe during the lengthy dilation stage? No one tells her. Women are simply left to terrible suffering.

But the answer is quite simple: she should not learn to breathe, but let the breathing come, as one does when practicing East Asian martial arts. She should breathe in the way described by the author Eugen Herrigel, who went to Japan in search of mystical experiences. In his marvelous little book *Zen in the Art of Archery,** which I cannot recommend highly enough to pregnant women, he describes how his master trained the students to breathe out slowly, regularly, and for as long as possible, accompanying their exhalation with a tone similar to the buzzing of a bee, thus enabling them to draw back the bow in a "relaxed" fashion.

This says it all. It is all about exhaling, even though people continue to talk only of breathing.

If something hits you, you cry out. This cry brings relief and is nothing other than a strongly ejected breath.

If you control your breathing, then everything changes. Once the buzzing of bees is replaced by a sonorous tone, you

---

*Eugen Herrigel, *Zen in the Art of Archery* (New York: Vintage, 1999).

can move into different spheres, especially when this tone is in harmony with the flawless sound of the tambūrā.

On this Indian stringed instrument, one does not play a melody; instead, as constantly and smoothly as possible, one repeats the fifth interval with the notes C and G, which corresponds to the most perfect harmony and serenity imaginable. This sound is the absolute rest and peace that Goethe declared to be perpetually present.

Now we come to practical matters.

Slow and regular exhalation is achieved only with the control of one's will; it can only arise from complete harmony with your movements, and your movements must emanate from this breathing. At some point, after continued practice, the breathing will happen as if by itself and will become one with your movements. The movement begins from a perfect-seated position, which is the position of Zazen, seated meditation: it can be done in the lotus or half-lotus position. What is necessary is that the knees should be rooted, as if to the ground.

But the woman can also sit in the Japanese manner, on her heels (possibly placing a small cushion between her heels and buttocks), making possible a gentle forward and backward movement. In doing this, her eyes should be constantly focused on the index finger of her right hand, which in a certain sense shows the direction, the way.

This seated position should not be assumed when

contractions begin. As long as the contractions are still endurable, the woman should walk up and down. She should never—absolutely never—lie in bed; she should not lie down at all. This degrades her and makes her into a sick person, when in fact she is steering her way toward the greatest joy in life.

This seated position, which leads to a perfect posture, free from any tension (to which Zen aspires), the Zazen position, should be assumed only when the contractions become very intense, very strong, indicating the end of cervical dilation, that is, the opening of the mouth of the uterus. These are the so-called good contractions, which in fact are absolutely unbearable and last a long time. Ten seconds? (Obstetricians, who see themselves as exact scientists, measure their duration with stopwatches.) Ten seconds is nothing. Twenty, thirty seconds? That is somewhat closer. Forty, fifty seconds? Now things get truly serious for the obstetrician, because all this is absolute hell for the woman.

It feels like hell because these contractions are, in fact, cramps. This means that the uterus is squeezing itself together as if to hold on to a prize that it doesn't want to release. The woman may have had cramps like this in her legs, but with a muscle as strong as the uterus, these cramps are awful.

The miracle—and it is a miracle—is that thanks to the breathing of Zazen, which is the breathing practiced in all East Asian martial arts (this fact cannot be repeated enough times), the woman can actually make herself have real contractions instead of these terrible cramps. With this breathing, the uterus no longer tightens up like a rock, but draws itself together slowly and gradually. At the end of the contraction there is a pause; this pause, very brief though it may be, is indispensable. Another gradual contraction follows, lasting the same amount of time, then there is another pause—and so one gentler contraction follows another.

What room is left for pain and suffering in this process? Ultimately, it all becomes simply a progression of sensations, which are as comfortable as . . . embraces.

A cooperation of movements, undulations, and breathing. Is that all?

Two things are of great importance here.

Firstly, you should never breathe into the upper chest area. This only releases feelings of anxiety. Correct breathing must come from the lower belly. The Japanese call it *hara* breathing.

Secondly, this breathing—or rather, this exhalation, this breathing out—should be accompanied by a tone, a musical note, which has revealed itself to be so effective in practicing.

Here two important elements play a decisive role: without this musical dimension, all the breathing remains only a bodily exercise, mere gymnastics. This is why it is so important to be in harmony with the tambūrā. The tone coming from this instrument may not seem to be all that special, but through the repetition of this C chord, which is also known as the perfect interval, it is in fact the embodiment of universal harmony, which transports the woman. This explains (if indeed an explanation is possible) her absolute inner peace, even in the middle of the most terrible storm. She feels completely secure.

The woman who practices singing and speaking the vowels as perfectly as possible in her preparatory exercises will be led to work very intensively with her lips and mouth, which also—mysteriously but unquestionably—has a definite effect on the cervix, which widens in a supremely harmonic and smooth manner under the influence of the exercises, at the very least making the contractions less painful.

Singing the Tones

"A" black
"I" red . . .

RIMBAUD

We now come to working on the tones, which is essential for preparation.

A, E, O, I, U, M

These are the tones that the woman must learn; basically, she must learn all over again how to pronounce them, how to voice them perfectly. This means she must articulate them and use all her ability to move her facial muscles. And she must learn to use the entire volume of her breath, until she has no more air left.

One can only give what one has received. To utter the tones correctly, you first need to experience them.

In the progress of this lesson, you are like a mirror. Go through the exercises without producing distorted images!

At the beginning, listen to the tambūrā.

Let its perfect tone pervade you, flow over you, take possession of you, and take off your corset. (You are very short of breath, without even knowing it.) Open yourself up wide.

Begin to open yourself as you are listening.

Now, only now, begin to work with the tone, to produce your own tone. This is not about singing. Instead it is an exercise that incorporates the entire human being, the whole person. For this reason it requires perfect posture, so that the formulation of the vowels and the emission of tones can take place in absolute harmony with your breathing and movements.

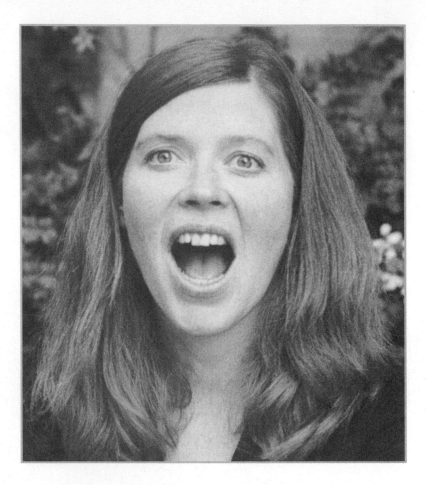

A

The *A* is the first letter of the alphabet, the first tone a child utters: Ma! Soon doubled, the tone is repeated like an echo: Mama! Papa!

But take care, your mouth must be open wide and this opening should not be a strain but should arise from a total relaxation of the face, expressing wonder and astonishment—not chomping down on your enthusiasm.

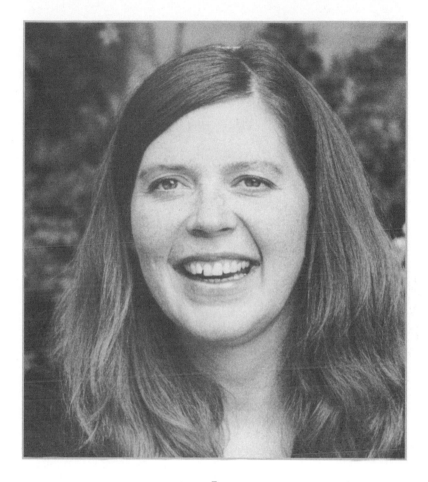

E

After the wide open *A*, which expresses deep contentment, the mouth now moves into a radiant smile. The ensuing *E* is truly <u>e</u>nchanting.

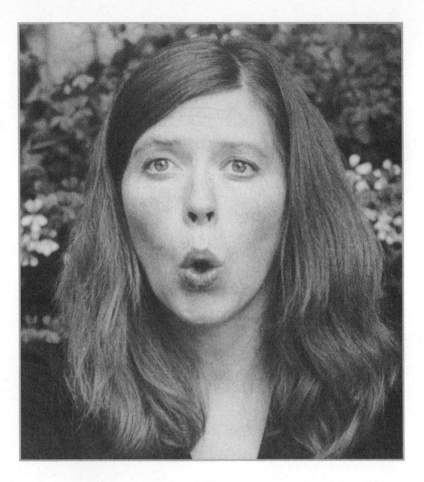

O

The mouth now changes from the passive or receiving position into action. The lips close again, forming a perfect small circle, a narrow opening, through which only a little air can escape. At the same time the eyebrows raise, as if expressing joyful surprise.

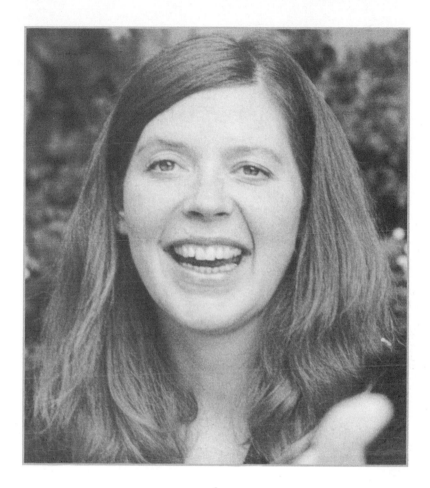

I

As the eyebrows lower again (the surprise is over), the mouth opens once more. The radiant smile returns. The *I* requires true exertion. This does not mean working the muscles strongly, but rather observing the expression. The corners of the mouth should be raised, making the smile genial, charming, and seductive.

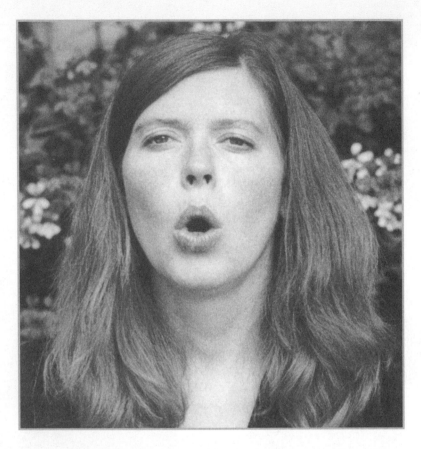

U

After this expressive demonstration of our ability, after we have greeted the outside world, we turn back inward, going to the source, to the silence with which everything began.

The mouth is half-closed, as if for a kiss, or as if one were about to whisper a secret. The eyebrows are also raised, as if requiring great attentiveness.

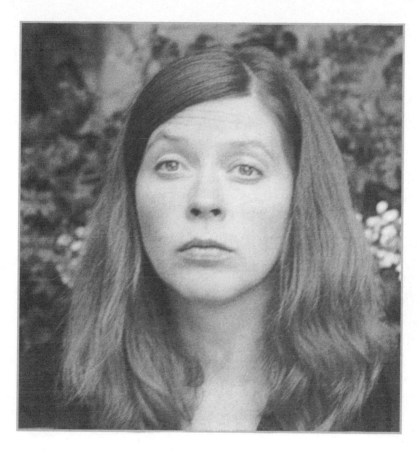

M

Now the mouth is closed again. But behind these closed lips, the teeth remain somewhat parted, so that the tone has a space for resonance, as much space as possible. This leads to a relaxation of the face, which is now entirely expressionless.

In this exercise, we have left the turbulent world of feelings behind us. Now we can finally dive back into silence.

During this stage, the liberated belly fills with air and empties as if by itself.

ABOUT THE EXERCISES

One more remark: What is meant by "attentiveness"? Here are a few tips on this, a few details:

Working with your mouth increases all your attentiveness. In breathing, the tone must be sustained for as long as possible, but only as long as it is comfortable. In addition, the tone must retain the same strength from beginning to end. The tone must never—really never—grow quieter or die away. This would mean that all the energy was leaking out of you, leaving you like a punctured tire. And here we come to the most important point:

As soon as the tone stops, as soon as there is no more air left, there is a pause, a break. During this pause, this interruption, in which you are totally relaxed, your belly (not your chest) will fill up and be prepared for the next exhalation. This pause is a great secret, especially since it takes place in such an enigmatic manner between all the contractions. Pausing means resting, even in the strongest storm. It alone will save you, otherwise shipwreck is unavoidable.

A final piece of advice: The emission of the tone goes exactly in parallel with movement forward from the back. This movement involves not only the hand but also the whole body, the whole being. One could say that it starts from the feet and then runs through the entire body, ending in the opposite hand.

It is a movement of complete continuity, appearing

through a forward inclination of the entire body, like a greeting. You bow as if to say: "Yes, My Lord."

When should the woman do these exercises?

Throughout pregnancy, as soon as the muse Euterpe has brushed her with her wings, but especially starting in the sixth month of pregnancy.

At what time of day should the exercises be practiced?

In the mornings, after bathing and eating breakfast.

How long should the exercises last?

Between ten minutes and half an hour. The most important thing is regularity. You can also do them in the evenings if you want.

Should the exercises be done during labor?

Only if the contractions are very long, strong, and painful.

What should one sing?

During pregnancy, sing the scale, quite simply, *C, D, E, F, G, A, B, C.* From bottom to top, then back down again.

Should one sing during labor?

What is good for the woman will naturally happen. The individual note will come to her: the note that corresponds to her personally, that allows her to say: "Yes, that's me!"—the note that will emerge from her exercises, or to use musical terminology, her keynote. This is the note that is connected to her life and comes from her heart.

What to do during the delivery stage?

The tone, a single tone, will come from her by itself.

ℐ

The exercises in this book appear in a modified form in my out-of-print book (accompanied by a cassette) *Atmen und Singen* [Breathing and Singing],* containing photos by Savitry Nayr. These photos further explain the facial expressions for the correct rendition and enunciation of the vowels *A, E, O, I, U,* and then, with the mouth closed, the consonant *M.* Here the entire work of breathing and toning is summarized. Savitry acquainted me with this way of working with the mouth and lips, namely diction, and I can also thank her for my having discovered the practically magical sound of the tambūrā. She was one of my greatest teachers, and for this I would like to pay her homage.

Our ways have now parted for various reasons. On the one hand, we were pursuing different goals: she taught singers, while I wanted to instruct women in a type of breathing that would enable them to change their experience of childbirth.

In any case, this led to the fact that this book is not illustrated by Savitry's photos, but by photos of a young woman who is a midwife herself. She has attended my seminars, passed the knowledge on, and enjoyed their good results herself (as she describes—see the letter from Stefanie S. in part 1). She is the best student of Raphaela Hoyer, who has also been mentioned earlier.

I was lucky to discover East Asian martial arts during

---

*Frédérick Leboyer, *Atmen und Singen. Einführung, Übungen. Mit einer Übungskassette von Savitry Nayr und Frédérick Leboyer zur "Kunst zu atmen"* (Munich: Kösel, 1984). Out of print.

my lifetime, first studying judo and aikido, then learning the incomparable art of tai chi chuan from a true master (not just a simple teacher or a good professor): the late Master Chil Kham, who died a few years ago at far too young an age. I pay homage to his memory here.

There are so many fine and various nuances in the perception of breathing. And breathing is anything but ordinary: thanks to it, every woman can remain captain of her ship as she sails through the storm.

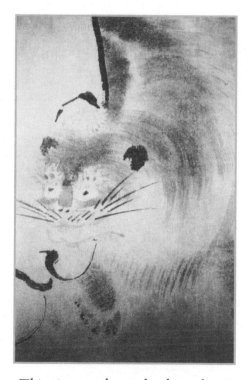

This tiger—what is he doing here?
He is the image of fear!
Look at him well!
Is he not smiling rather charmingly?

Using the CD

The CD includes singing exercises to the sound of the tambūrā as well as the sound of the tambūrā solo. Both are live recordings.

> **Track 1.** Singing exercises to the sound of the tambūrā (6:00 min.)
> **Track 2.** The sound of the tambūrā solo (20:48 min.)

DURING PREGNANCY

Especially after the sixth month of pregnancy, or earlier if desired, depending on your personal needs.

First: Listen to the sound of the tambūrā, then to the singing, but without singing yourself. Just listen with all your attention!

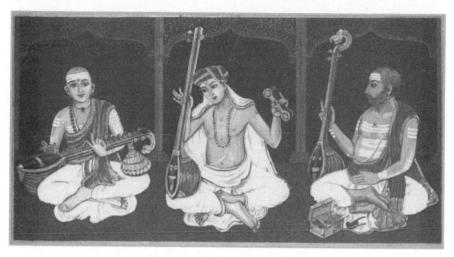

TAMBŪRĀ IN CENTER

Second: Play the CD again, from the beginning. But this time try toning along with the singers.

Third, and this is the most important and useful thing for you: Go directly to the second part of the CD (track 2), on which you can hear the sound of the tambūrā by itself. Forget all about the singing. First, just listen to the sound of the tambūrā and let a tone, a note, come out of you entirely spontaneously. Make sure the tone is comfortable for you and doesn't cause you any strain.

Then, repeat this note again and again, until you are entirely sure and have the feeling: "Oh, yes, that's me!"

With this, you have found your own personal tone. This is a great achievement.

DURING LABOR

When you are in labor and the contractions are growing stronger, begin singing your own tone, again and again, but always to the sound of the tambūrā.

You should *not* sing the entire exercise, not the complete scale, but only your own entirely personal tone.

This will save you.

The strong contractions at the end of the dilation stage, when the mouth of the uterus opens, cause intense cramps. The uterus draws itself together very tightly and does not want to let go. It remains contracted and as hard as rock, which is very painful.

When you sing your own tone to the sound of the tambūrā, these terrible cramps will vanish. Your uterus will stop pulling itself inward so forcefully, but instead much more slowly, and then gradually, after a short (and necessary) pause (this pause is very important and should under no circumstances be lacking), the cramp will release and the uterus will relax, very slowly.

Now true contractions and not cramps follow, and therefore no more pain.

All women who have completed this training and sung to the sound of the tambūrā—really all of them—have said that it was the lifeboat that saved them from the storm of labor.

Photo Credits

About the Author

Born in France in 1918, Frédérick Leboyer graduated from the University of Paris School of Medicine, where he later became Chef de Clinique in the 1950s. During his time as an obstetrician, he attended more than ten thousand births. He became increasingly dissatisfied with the impersonal clinical treatment of the newborn child and began working on new ideas about the process of birth. This reassessment resulted in his groundbreaking *Birth without Violence,* first published in France in 1974. This book revolutionized the course of prenatal care and the way babies are introduced into the world.

Frédérick Leboyer first visited India in 1959 and spent two months a year there in the following two decades. He developed a deep interest in yoga and its applications to pregnancy and childbirth, especially in the use of breathing and sound. He found that by using the music of the tambūrā, the Indian stringed instrument whose tone represents the embodiment of universal harmony, that women could be transported to a place of deep inner peace—a place of rest and harmony useful during both pregnancy and the labor of birth.

Three years after the publication of *Birth without Violence,* Leboyer wrote *Loving Hands,* a book inspired by his observation in Calcutta of a young mother named Shantala lovingly massaging her baby. In her honor, Leboyer gave her name to this form of massage.

Frédérick Leboyer is credited as the founder of the modern gentle birth movement. Since retiring from his medical practice, Leboyer has conducted worldwide seminars and workshops for pregnant women, midwives, gynecologists, and pediatricians. He lives in Switzerland.

BOOKS OF RELATED INTEREST

Birth without Violence
by Frédérick Leboyer, M.D.

Gentle Birth Choices
by Barbara Harper, R.N.

The Edison Gene
ADHD and the Gift of the Hunter Child
by Thom Hartmann

Vaccinations: A Thoughtful Parent's Guide
How to Make Safe, Sensible Decisions about the
Risks, Benefits, and Alternatives
by Aviva Jill Romm

Natural Health after Birth
The Complete Guide to Postpartum Wellness
by Aviva Jill Romm

Parenting Begins Before Conception
A Guide to Preparing Body, Mind, and Spirit for
You and Your Future Child
by Carista Luminare-Rosen, Ph.D.

Labor Pain
A Natural Approach to Easing Delivery
by Nicky Wesson

Reclaiming the Spirituality of Birth
Healing for Mothers and Babies
by Benig Mauger

INNER TRADITIONS • BEAR & COMPANY
P.O. Box 388
Rochester, VT 05767
1-800-246-8648
www.InnerTraditions.com
Or contact your local bookseller